NAVIGATING THE USAGE OF POSTINOR-2

THE COMPREHENSIVE GUIDE ON THE EMERGENCY CONTRACEPTIVE

TABLE OF CONTENTS

CHAPTER 1 4

INTRODUCTION TO POSTINOR-2 4

1.1 Overview of Emergency Contraception 4

1.2 What is Postinor-2? 5

1.3 History and Development..6

1.4 Importance and Relevance 7

CHAPTER 2 10

HOW POSTINOR-2 WORKS.......................................10

2.1 Mechanism of Action 10

2.2 Effectiveness 11

2.3 Time Frame for Usage..13

CHAPTER 3 16

USAGE GUIDELINES..16

3.1 Indications for Use 16

3.2 Dosage Instructions 17

3.3 How to Take Postinor-2 18

3.4 What to Do If You Vomit After Taking Postinor-2
....20

Additional Considerations...21

CHAPTER 4 23

SIDE EFFECTS AND SAFETY 23

4.1 Common Side Effects..23

4.2 Rare but Serious Side Effects...............................24

4.3 Contraindications..26

4.4 Interactions with Other Medications 27

4.5 Safety Considerations.....................................28

CHAPTER 5 31

FREQUENTLY ASKED QUESTIONS 31

5.1 What Happens If You Take Postinor-2 Multiple Times? 31

5.2 Can Postinor-2 Affect Future Fertility?................32

5.3 Is Postinor-2 Effective During Ovulation?...........33

5.4 What Are the Alternatives to Postinor-2? 35

5.5 How to Access Postinor-2 36

Final Considerations..38

CHAPTER 6 40

CONCLUSION 40

6.1 Summary of Key Points 40

6.2 Final Recommendations 43

CHAPTER 1

INTRODUCTION TO POSTINOR-2

1.1 Overview of Emergency Contraception

Emergency contraception (EC) refers to the methods used to prevent pregnancy after unprotected sexual intercourse or contraceptive failure, such as a broken condom or missed birth control pills. It is a crucial option for preventing unintended pregnancies and is an important aspect of reproductive health. EC methods are designed to be used shortly after intercourse and are not intended as regular birth control methods. They provide a vital safety net for individuals who experience contraceptive mishaps or have unprotected sex.

There are primarily two types of emergency contraception: emergency contraceptive pills (ECPs) and the copper intrauterine device (IUD). ECPs are divided into two main categories: those containing levonorgestrel (like Postinor-2) and those containing ulipristal acetate (such as Ella). The copper IUD is a non-hormonal option that can be used up to five days after unprotected intercourse and provides ongoing contraception for up to ten years if left in place.

Levonorgestrel-based emergency contraceptive pills, like Postinor-2, are among the most commonly used EC methods due to their availability, effectiveness, and ease of use. They are typically available over-the-counter in many countries, making them accessible to individuals in need of urgent contraception. Understanding the role and proper use of these methods is essential for those seeking to prevent unintended pregnancies effectively.

1.2 What is Postinor-2?

Postinor-2 is a widely used emergency contraceptive pill that contains the active ingredient levonorgestrel, a synthetic progestogen. It is designed to prevent pregnancy when taken within a specific time frame after unprotected intercourse. The name "Postinor" suggests its use after an event (post) to prevent the beginning of a pregnancy.

Each Postinor-2 pack contains two pills, each with 0.75 mg of levonorgestrel. The standard regimen involves taking the first pill as soon as possible after unprotected sex, followed by the second pill 12 hours later. Alternatively, both pills can be taken together as a single dose, depending on the recommendation provided in the specific region or country.

Levonorgestrel works primarily by inhibiting ovulation, the release of an egg from the ovary. It may also prevent fertilization by affecting the movement of sperm and egg through the fallopian tubes or alter the lining of the uterus to prevent implantation of a fertilized egg. It is important to note that Postinor-2 is not effective if implantation has already occurred, and it does not terminate an existing pregnancy.

1.3 History and Development

The development of Postinor-2 is part of the broader history of emergency contraception, which has evolved significantly over the past few decades. The concept of postcoital contraception dates back to the 1960s when researchers began exploring high doses of oral contraceptives to prevent pregnancy after unprotected sex. Early methods involved using combinations of estrogen and progestin, which were effective but often associated with significant side effects such as nausea and vomiting.

In the 1970s and 1980s, the Yuzpe regimen, which combined high doses of estrogen and progestin, became a widely recognized method of emergency contraception.

However, the search for more effective and tolerable options continued. Researchers began to focus on levonorgestrel, a synthetic progestogen, as a potential candidate for emergency contraception due to its high efficacy and lower incidence of side effects.

In the late 1990s, clinical trials demonstrated that levonorgestrel-alone regimens were as effective, if not more so, than the Yuzpe regimen, with fewer side effects. This led to the development and approval of levonorgestrel-based emergency contraceptives, including Postinor-2. The simplicity and effectiveness of a progestin-only regimen made it a preferred choice for many healthcare providers and individuals seeking emergency contraception.

Since its introduction, Postinor-2 has been widely adopted in many countries, becoming a key option in reproductive health care. Its over-the-counter availability in numerous regions has further enhanced its accessibility, empowering individuals to take control of their reproductive health in urgent situations.

1.4 Importance and Relevance

The importance and relevance of Postinor-2 in contemporary reproductive health cannot be overstated. Unintended pregnancies can have significant social, economic, and health implications for individuals and communities. Access to effective emergency contraception like Postinor-2 is crucial in reducing the incidence of unintended pregnancies and providing individuals with the means to make informed decisions about their reproductive health.

Postinor-2 plays a critical role in several scenarios:

1. **Contraceptive Failure:** Even with regular use of contraception, failures can occur. Condoms can break, and birth control pills can be missed. Postinor-2 provides a safety net in such instances, helping to prevent an unintended pregnancy.

2. **Unprotected Intercourse:** In cases of unprotected sex, whether due to lack of access to contraception, coercion, or unplanned encounters, Postinor-2 offers a reliable option to prevent pregnancy.

3. **Sexual Assault:** For survivors of sexual assault, access to emergency contraception is a vital aspect of post-assault care. Postinor-2 can provide immediate relief

and control over their reproductive choices in a difficult time.

4. **Accessibility and Empowerment:** The over-the-counter availability of Postinor-2 in many regions means that individuals do not require a prescription, thereby reducing barriers to access. This empowers individuals, especially women, to take proactive steps in managing their reproductive health.

5. **Public Health Impact:** By preventing unintended pregnancies, Postinor-2 contributes to better health outcomes for women and families. It helps in reducing the number of unsafe abortions and associated complications, which are significant public health concerns in many parts of the world.

CHAPTER 2

HOW POSTINOR-2 WORKS

2.1 Mechanism of Action

Postinor-2, an emergency contraceptive pill containing the active ingredient levonorgestrel, functions through multiple mechanisms to prevent pregnancy. Understanding these mechanisms is crucial to comprehending how Postinor-2 provides effective emergency contraception.

Inhibition of Ovulation: The primary mechanism by which Postinor-2 works is by inhibiting or delaying ovulation. Ovulation is the process during which an ovary releases an egg (ovum) into the fallopian tube, where it can potentially be fertilized by sperm. Levonorgestrel, the synthetic progestogen in Postinor-2, interferes with the normal hormonal signals that trigger ovulation. By altering the surge of luteinizing hormone (LH) that precedes ovulation, Postinor-2 can prevent the ovary from releasing an egg. If there is no egg available for fertilization, pregnancy cannot occur.

Alteration of Cervical Mucus: Postinor-2 also affects the cervical mucus, making it thicker and more viscous. This change in the cervical mucus creates a barrier that impedes sperm movement, making it more difficult for sperm to travel through the cervix and reach the egg. By hindering sperm motility and preventing their passage through the reproductive tract, Postinor-2 reduces the likelihood of fertilization.

Changes to the Endometrium: Another potential mechanism is the alteration of the endometrium, the lining of the uterus. Levonorgestrel may cause changes to the endometrial lining, making it less receptive to the implantation of a fertilized egg. If fertilization were to occur, the altered endometrial environment could prevent the implantation and subsequent development of the embryo. However, it is important to note that Postinor-2 is not effective if implantation has already taken place, as it does not induce abortion or harm an existing pregnancy.

2.2 Effectiveness

The effectiveness of Postinor-2 as an emergency contraceptive is well-documented, although its efficacy depends on various factors, including the timing of administration and the individual's menstrual cycle.

Timing of Administration: The effectiveness of Postinor-2 is highest when taken as soon as possible after unprotected intercourse. Studies have shown that when taken within 24 hours of unprotected sex, Postinor-2 can reduce the risk of pregnancy by up to 95%. If taken within 48 hours, the effectiveness remains high, but it begins to decline, with an estimated effectiveness of around 85%. When taken within 72 hours, the effectiveness is approximately 58-95%, depending on the study and the specific circumstances. Thus, prompt administration is crucial for maximizing its efficacy.

Menstrual Cycle Phase: The phase of the menstrual cycle during which Postinor-2 is taken can also influence its effectiveness. If taken before ovulation, Postinor-2 is more likely to prevent the release of an egg, thereby preventing fertilization. If taken after ovulation, the effectiveness may be reduced because the primary mechanism of inhibiting ovulation is no longer applicable. However, Postinor-2 may still exert its effects by altering cervical mucus and the endometrial lining.

Body Weight and BMI: Emerging research suggests that body weight and body mass index (BMI) may impact the effectiveness of levonorgestrel-based emergency contraceptives like Postinor-2. Some studies have indicated that higher body weight or BMI might reduce the efficacy of these pills. While further research is needed to confirm these findings, individuals with higher BMI may want to consider alternative emergency contraceptive methods, such as the copper IUD, for more reliable protection.

Recurrent Use: It is important to note that Postinor-2 is intended for occasional use and not as a regular contraceptive method. Repeated use within a single menstrual cycle may result in diminished effectiveness and increased side effects. Individuals who find themselves frequently relying on emergency contraception should consult a healthcare provider to discuss more suitable long-term contraceptive options.

2.3 Time Frame for Usage

The time frame for using Postinor-2 is a critical aspect of its effectiveness. Understanding the optimal and permissible windows for administration is essential for ensuring maximum efficacy.

Optimal Time Frame: The optimal time frame for taking Postinor-2 is as soon as possible after unprotected intercourse. Ideally, it should be taken within 24 hours, as this time frame provides the highest level of effectiveness. Prompt action is crucial because the sooner the pill is taken, the more likely it is to prevent ovulation and reduce the risk of pregnancy.

Permissible Time Frame: While the optimal window is within 24 hours, Postinor-2 can still be effective if taken within 72 hours (three days) of unprotected sex. The effectiveness gradually decreases with each passing hour, but it remains a viable option for preventing pregnancy up to the 72-hour mark. Beyond 72 hours, the efficacy of Postinor-2 is significantly reduced, and alternative emergency contraception methods should be considered, such as the copper IUD, which can be effective up to five days after unprotected intercourse.

Administration Instructions: Postinor-2 is typically administered in a two-pill regimen. The first pill should be taken as soon as possible after unprotected sex, followed by the second pill 12 hours later. However, in some regions, a single-dose regimen may be recommended, where both pills are taken together at once. It is important to follow the specific instructions provided with the product or those given by a healthcare provider.

Delayed Administration: If there is a delay in taking Postinor-2 beyond the 72-hour window, it is advisable to seek guidance from a healthcare professional. While Postinor-2 may still offer some protection, its effectiveness is considerably diminished, and other emergency contraception options should be explored.

Factors Influencing Timing: Several factors can influence the timing and effectiveness of Postinor-2. These include the timing of unprotected sex in relation to the menstrual cycle, the individual's body weight and BMI, and any potential interactions with other medications. It is essential to consider these factors when determining the appropriate use of Postinor-2.

CHAPTER 3

USAGE GUIDELINES

3.1 Indications for Use

Postinor-2 is an emergency contraceptive pill designed to prevent pregnancy after unprotected sexual intercourse or contraceptive failure. It is not intended for regular use and should only be used in specific circumstances where immediate contraception is necessary.

Unprotected Intercourse: Postinor-2 is indicated for use after unprotected sex, which can occur for various reasons. This includes instances where no contraceptive method was used, a contraceptive method was used incorrectly (such as missing birth control pills), or a condom broke or slipped off during intercourse. It is also useful in cases where a diaphragm or contraceptive sponge was not placed properly or fell out.

Contraceptive Failure: Even with the regular use of contraceptives, failures can happen. For example, a condom may break, or a woman may forget to take her regular contraceptive pills. In such cases, Postinor-2 provides a backup option to prevent unintended pregnancy.

Sexual Assault: Postinor-2 is also indicated for use by survivors of sexual assault who are at risk of becoming pregnant as a result of the assault. Access to emergency contraception is a critical component of post-assault care, helping to provide control over reproductive health during a traumatic time.

It is important to note that Postinor-2 is not an abortion pill and does not work if a woman is already pregnant. It is also not intended to replace regular contraceptive methods and should not be used as a primary form of birth control. Individuals who find themselves needing emergency contraception frequently should consult with a healthcare provider to discuss more reliable and consistent contraceptive options.

3.2 Dosage Instructions

Postinor-2 is typically available in a pack containing two pills, each with 0.75 mg of levonorgestrel. The dosage instructions are straightforward but must be followed precisely to ensure maximum effectiveness.

Standard Regimen: The standard regimen involves taking the first pill as soon as possible after unprotected sex, followed by the second pill 12 hours later. This two-dose regimen ensures that the active ingredient, levonorgestrel, is maintained at effective levels in the body to prevent pregnancy.

Single-Dose Regimen: In some regions, a single-dose regimen is recommended, where both pills are taken together as a single dose. This approach simplifies the administration process and ensures that the full dose is taken at once, reducing the risk of forgetting the second dose.

Regardless of the regimen, it is critical to take Postinor-2 as soon as possible after unprotected sex. The sooner it is taken, the more effective it will be in preventing pregnancy.

3.3 How to Take Postinor-2

Taking Postinor-2 correctly is essential for its effectiveness. Here are detailed steps on how to take Postinor-2:

Step 1: Obtain Postinor-2: Postinor-2 is available over-the-counter in many countries, so it can be purchased from pharmacies without a prescription. Ensure that you have a pack of Postinor-2 that is within its expiration date.

Step 2: Take the First Pill: If using the standard two-dose regimen, take the first pill as soon as possible after unprotected sex. The pill should be swallowed whole with water. Do not crush or chew the pill, as this could affect its absorption and effectiveness.

Step 3: Take the Second Pill: If following the standard regimen, take the second pill 12 hours after the first one. It is crucial to adhere to this timing to ensure the highest level of effectiveness. Set a reminder if necessary to avoid missing the second dose.

Step 4: Single-Dose Option: If the single-dose regimen is recommended in your region, take both pills together at the same time. This simplifies the process and ensures that the full dose is taken at once.

Step 5: Monitor for Side Effects: After taking Postinor-2, monitor for any side effects. Common side effects may include nausea, fatigue, headache, dizziness, breast tenderness, and changes in menstrual bleeding. These side effects are usually mild and temporary.

3.4 What to Do If You Vomit After Taking Postinor-2

Vomiting after taking Postinor-2 can affect its effectiveness because the active ingredient, levonorgestrel, may not be fully absorbed into the bloodstream. If vomiting occurs, it is important to take appropriate steps to ensure that the emergency contraception is effective.

Within 2 Hours: If vomiting occurs within two hours of taking either the first or second pill, it is likely that the pill has not been fully absorbed. In this case, you should take another dose as soon as possible. This means taking an additional pill to replace the one that was vomited out. If you do not have an extra pack of Postinor-2, you should obtain another one from a pharmacy or healthcare provider immediately.

After 2 Hours: If vomiting occurs more than two hours after taking the pill, the active ingredient has likely been absorbed sufficiently, and you do not need to take another dose. However, if you are unsure or concerned about the effectiveness of the medication, consult with a healthcare provider for further advice.

Persistent Vomiting: If you continue to experience vomiting or severe nausea, it may be challenging to keep the medication down. In such cases, seek medical advice. A healthcare provider may recommend an anti-nausea medication to help keep the contraceptive pill down or may suggest an alternative method of emergency contraception, such as the copper IUD.

Alternative Methods: If vomiting is severe and persistent, and you are unable to take Postinor-2 effectively, consider using an alternative form of emergency contraception. The copper IUD is a highly effective option that can be inserted by a healthcare provider up to five days after unprotected sex. It provides immediate and ongoing contraception and is not affected by vomiting.

Additional Considerations

Menstrual Changes: After taking Postinor-2, some women may experience changes in their menstrual cycle. Your next period may come earlier or later than expected, and the flow may be lighter or heavier than usual. These changes are generally temporary and should normalize in the following cycle. If your period is more than a week late, it is advisable to take a pregnancy test to rule out pregnancy.

Interactions with Other Medications: Certain medications can interact with Postinor-2 and affect its effectiveness. These include some antiepileptic drugs, antibiotics, and herbal supplements like St. John's Wort. If you are taking any other medications, inform your healthcare provider or pharmacist before using Postinor-2 to ensure there are no interactions that could reduce its efficacy.

Long-Term Contraception: Postinor-2 is not intended for regular use as a contraceptive method. It is designed for occasional, emergency situations. If you find yourself needing emergency contraception frequently, it is important to consult with a healthcare provider to discuss more reliable and consistent methods of birth control, such as oral contraceptives, intrauterine devices (IUDs), implants, or contraceptive injections.

CHAPTER 4

SIDE EFFECTS AND SAFETY

4.1 Common Side Effects

Like all medications, Postinor-2 can cause side effects, although not everyone experiences them. Most side effects associated with Postinor-2 are mild and temporary. Understanding these potential side effects can help users prepare and manage them effectively.

Nausea and Vomiting: One of the most common side effects of Postinor-2 is nausea, which can sometimes lead to vomiting. This is due to the high dose of levonorgestrel, which can irritate the stomach. If vomiting occurs within two hours of taking the pill, it may be necessary to take another dose to ensure effectiveness.

Fatigue: Many users report feeling tired or fatigued after taking Postinor-2. This is typically short-lived and should resolve within a day or two.

Headache: Headaches are another common side effect. Over-the-counter pain relievers, such as ibuprofen or acetaminophen, can help alleviate this symptom.

Dizziness: Some individuals may experience dizziness or lightheadedness after taking Postinor-2. Staying hydrated and resting can help manage these symptoms.

Breast Tenderness: Hormonal fluctuations caused by levonorgestrel can lead to breast tenderness or discomfort. This side effect usually subsides within a few days.

Menstrual Changes: Postinor-2 can cause changes in the menstrual cycle. The next period may be earlier or later than expected, and the flow may be lighter or heavier. These changes are generally temporary and should normalize in subsequent cycles.

Abdominal Pain: Mild abdominal or pelvic pain can occur after taking Postinor-2. This is typically not severe and should resolve on its own.

4.2 Rare but Serious Side Effects

While most side effects of Postinor-2 are mild, there are rare but serious side effects that users should be aware of. If any of these occur, it is important to seek medical attention immediately.

Severe Abdominal Pain: Although mild abdominal pain is common, severe pain could indicate a more serious condition such as an ectopic pregnancy (where a fertilized egg implants outside the uterus). This is a medical emergency and requires prompt treatment.

Allergic Reactions: In rare cases, individuals may experience an allergic reaction to levonorgestrel. Symptoms of an allergic reaction include rash, itching, swelling (especially of the face, tongue, or throat), severe dizziness, and difficulty breathing. An allergic reaction to Postinor-2 necessitates immediate medical attention.

Severe Headaches or Migraine: While headaches are common, severe headaches or migraines can occur in rare instances. If the headache is accompanied by visual disturbances, nausea, or vomiting, medical advice should be sought.

Chest Pain or Shortness of Breath: Although extremely rare, chest pain or shortness of breath after taking Postinor-2 could indicate a cardiovascular issue. Immediate medical evaluation is necessary in such cases.

Jaundice: Yellowing of the skin or eyes (jaundice) is a rare side effect that may indicate liver issues. This requires prompt medical attention.

4.3 Contraindications

Certain conditions and circumstances may contraindicate the use of Postinor-2. It is important for individuals to be aware of these contraindications and consult with a healthcare provider if any of these apply.

Pregnancy: Postinor-2 is not effective if a woman is already pregnant and should not be used as an abortifacient. It does not harm an existing pregnancy, but it will not prevent an ongoing pregnancy.

Hypersensitivity: Individuals with known hypersensitivity or allergy to levonorgestrel or any other component of Postinor-2 should not use this medication.

Severe Liver Disease: Women with severe liver impairment should avoid using Postinor-2, as the medication is metabolized by the liver. In such cases, alternative emergency contraceptive methods should be considered.

Unexplained Vaginal Bleeding: Women experiencing unexplained vaginal bleeding should seek medical evaluation before using Postinor-2 to rule out underlying conditions that may require different treatment.

4.4 Interactions with Other Medications

Certain medications and substances can interact with Postinor-2, potentially reducing its effectiveness or increasing the risk of side effects. It is important to inform healthcare providers of all medications and supplements being taken to identify any potential interactions.

Enzyme Inducers: Medications that induce liver enzymes (such as certain antiepileptic drugs, rifampicin, rifabutin, and some antiretroviral drugs) can increase the metabolism of levonorgestrel, reducing its effectiveness. St. John's Wort, a herbal supplement, can also have this effect. Women taking these medications may need to consider alternative forms of emergency contraception.

Certain Antibiotics: While most antibiotics do not interact with hormonal contraceptives, antibiotics like rifampicin and rifabutin, which are enzyme inducers, can reduce the effectiveness of Postinor-2.

Grapefruit Juice: Grapefruit juice can increase the levels of levonorgestrel in the blood, potentially increasing the risk of side effects. It is advisable to avoid consuming grapefruit juice while using Postinor-2.

4.5 Safety Considerations Overall, Postinor-2 is considered safe for most women when used as directed. However, certain safety considerations should be kept in mind to ensure its effective and safe use.

Frequency of Use: Postinor-2 is intended for occasional use and should not be used as a regular form of contraception. Frequent use can lead to increased side effects and reduced effectiveness. Women who find themselves needing emergency contraception frequently should consult with a healthcare provider to discuss more reliable long-term contraceptive options.

Body Weight and BMI: Emerging research suggests that body weight and BMI may affect the effectiveness of levonorgestrel-based emergency contraception. Women with higher body weight or BMI may have reduced effectiveness. In such cases, alternative emergency contraceptive methods, like the copper IUD, may be more effective.

Menstrual Cycle Monitoring: After taking Postinor-2, women should monitor their menstrual cycle. While some changes are expected, a significantly delayed period (more than a week late) may indicate pregnancy. In such cases, a pregnancy test should be taken, and medical advice should be sought.

Breastfeeding: Postinor-2 is generally considered safe for use during breastfeeding. Levonorgestrel passes into breast milk in small amounts, but it is not expected to harm a breastfeeding infant. However, if there are any concerns, women should consult with a healthcare provider.

Age Considerations: Postinor-2 is approved for use in women of reproductive age, including adolescents. However, younger women, especially those under 16, should seek guidance from a healthcare provider to ensure they receive appropriate support and follow-up care.

Healthcare Consultation: While Postinor-2 is available over-the-counter in many regions, consulting with a healthcare provider can provide valuable information and support. A healthcare provider can help assess individual risk factors, discuss potential interactions with other medications, and provide guidance on the most appropriate and effective use of emergency contraception.

Storage and Handling: Postinor-2 should be stored at room temperature, away from direct sunlight and moisture. It should be kept out of reach of children. Proper storage ensures the medication remains effective until its expiration date.

CHAPTER 5

FREQUENTLY ASKED QUESTIONS

5.1 What Happens If You Take Postinor-2 Multiple Times?

Using Postinor-2 more than once is a concern for many women who may find themselves in repeated situations where emergency contraception is needed. While it is generally safe to use Postinor-2 multiple times, there are important considerations to keep in mind.

Safety and Side Effects: Taking Postinor-2 multiple times is not associated with any long-term health risks or serious complications. However, frequent use can lead to more pronounced side effects. Common side effects such as nausea, fatigue, headache, and menstrual irregularities may become more noticeable with repeated use.

Menstrual Irregularities: One of the most significant impacts of using Postinor-2 multiple times is on the menstrual cycle. Women may experience irregular bleeding, spotting, or changes in the timing and flow of their periods. These disruptions can make it difficult to predict the menstrual cycle and may cause anxiety.

Effectiveness: While Postinor-2 is effective at preventing pregnancy after unprotected sex, it is less effective than regular contraceptive methods when used repeatedly. The efficacy of Postinor-2 can decrease with frequent use, making it a less reliable form of contraception over time.

Long-Term Contraception: Postinor-2 is designed for emergency situations and is not intended to be used as a regular form of birth control. Women who find themselves needing emergency contraception frequently should consider more reliable long-term contraceptive options. Methods such as oral contraceptives, intrauterine devices (IUDs), contraceptive implants, or injectable contraceptives provide more consistent and effective protection against pregnancy.

5.2 Can Postinor-2 Affect Future Fertility?

A common concern among women is whether the use of Postinor-2 can impact their future fertility. The good news is that Postinor-2 does not have any long-term effects on fertility.

Temporary Effects: While Postinor-2 can cause temporary disruptions in the menstrual cycle, these changes are generally short-lived and should resolve within a few cycles. Any irregularities in bleeding or changes in the timing of periods are usually temporary and do not affect long-term reproductive health.

Return to Fertility: Fertility returns to normal quickly after the use of Postinor-2. Women who have used Postinor-2 and wish to conceive can expect their fertility to return to its baseline level almost immediately. There is no evidence to suggest that Postinor-2 has any lasting impact on a woman's ability to conceive in the future.

No Impact on Ovarian Function: Postinor-2 works primarily by preventing or delaying ovulation. It does not cause any permanent changes to ovarian function or damage to the reproductive organs. Once the effects of the medication wear off, the ovaries continue to function normally.

5.3 Is Postinor-2 Effective During Ovulation?

The effectiveness of Postinor-2 depends on the timing of administration relative to the menstrual cycle. Ovulation is a critical phase, and many women wonder if Postinor-2 is effective if taken during ovulation.

Mechanism of Action: Postinor-2 works by inhibiting or delaying ovulation. If taken before ovulation occurs, it can effectively prevent the release of an egg, thus preventing fertilization. However, if ovulation has already occurred, Postinor-2 may be less effective because its primary mechanism of action is no longer applicable.

Limited Effectiveness Post-Ovulation: If a woman is already ovulating or has recently ovulated, Postinor-2 may not be able to prevent fertilization effectively. In such cases, the efficacy of Postinor-2 is reduced. While it may still alter the cervical mucus and endometrial lining to some extent, these mechanisms are less reliable in preventing pregnancy once ovulation has occurred.

Alternative Options: For women who are concerned about the timing of ovulation, the copper IUD is a highly effective alternative. The copper IUD can be inserted up to five days after unprotected intercourse and is effective regardless of the timing of ovulation. It provides ongoing contraception for up to 10 years.

5.4 What Are the Alternatives to Postinor-2?

While Postinor-2 is a widely used emergency contraceptive, there are several alternative methods available for preventing pregnancy after unprotected sex or contraceptive failure.

Copper IUD: The copper IUD (intrauterine device) is the most effective form of emergency contraception. It can be inserted by a healthcare provider up to five days after unprotected intercourse. The copper IUD works by creating an inhospitable environment for sperm and eggs, preventing fertilization and implantation. It also provides long-term contraception for up to 10 years.

Ulipristal Acetate (Ella): Ulipristal acetate, sold under the brand name Ella, is another emergency contraceptive pill. It is a selective progesterone receptor modulator that can be taken up to five days after unprotected sex. Ella is more effective than levonorgestrel-based pills like Postinor-2, especially if taken closer to the time of ovulation.

Regular Birth Control Pills: In some cases, certain combinations of regular birth control pills can be used as emergency contraception. This method, known as the Yuzpe regimen, involves taking a higher dose of regular birth control pills in two doses, 12 hours apart. However, this method is less effective and more likely to cause side effects compared to dedicated emergency contraceptive pills.

Progestin-Only Pills: Higher doses of regular progestin-only birth control pills can also be used for emergency contraception. Like the Yuzpe regimen, this method is less effective and can cause more side effects than dedicated emergency contraceptive pills.

5.5 How to Access Postinor-2

Access to Postinor-2 varies by region, but it is generally available over-the-counter in many countries. Here are some common ways to obtain Postinor-2:

Pharmacies: In many countries, Postinor-2 can be purchased without a prescription at pharmacies. Pharmacists can provide information on how to use the medication and answer any questions. Some pharmacies may also offer confidential consultations to discuss emergency contraception options.

Online Purchase: Postinor-2 can often be purchased online from reputable pharmacies. This option provides convenience and privacy, allowing individuals to order the medication discreetly and have it delivered to their home. It is important to ensure that the online pharmacy is legitimate and that the medication is genuine.

Health Clinics: Many health clinics, including family planning clinics and sexual health centers, provide emergency contraception. These clinics often offer confidential services and can provide Postinor-2 along with information on other contraceptive options.

Healthcare Providers: Women can also obtain Postinor-2 from their healthcare providers. Doctors, nurse practitioners, and other healthcare professionals can prescribe and dispense emergency contraception. Consulting with a healthcare provider can provide an opportunity to discuss long-term contraceptive options and receive personalized advice.

Emergency Rooms: In cases of sexual assault or other emergencies, Postinor-2 may be available at hospital emergency rooms. Healthcare providers in these settings can offer immediate care and support, including providing emergency contraception.

Community Programs: Some community health programs and non-profit organizations provide free or low-cost emergency contraception to those in need. These programs aim to increase access to emergency contraception for individuals who may face financial or other barriers.

Age Restrictions: In some regions, there may be age restrictions on the purchase of Postinor-2. Younger individuals, especially those under the age of 16, may need to obtain a prescription or consult with a healthcare provider to access emergency contraception.

Final Considerations

Timely Access: Regardless of the method of obtaining Postinor-2, it is crucial to take the medication as soon as possible after unprotected sex to maximize its effectiveness. Delays in obtaining and taking the medication can reduce its ability to prevent pregnancy.

Storage: Postinor-2 should be stored at room temperature, away from direct sunlight and moisture. Keeping a pack of Postinor-2 on hand can ensure timely access in case of an emergency.

Education and Awareness: Increasing awareness and education about emergency contraception options can help individuals make informed decisions about their reproductive health. Healthcare providers, educators, and community organizations play a vital role in providing accurate information and support.

CHAPTER 6

CONCLUSION

6.1 Summary of Key Points

Emergency contraception is a critical component of reproductive healthcare, providing a last-resort option to prevent pregnancy after unprotected sex or contraceptive failure. Postinor-2, a popular emergency contraceptive, has been widely used for its effectiveness and accessibility. Understanding its use, effectiveness, side effects, and safety is essential for making informed decisions about reproductive health.

Overview of Emergency Contraception: Emergency contraception, including Postinor-2, offers a way to prevent pregnancy after unprotected sex. It should not be confused with abortion pills; instead, it prevents fertilization or implantation if taken within a specific time frame.

What is Postinor-2?: Postinor-2 contains levonorgestrel, a synthetic hormone that helps prevent pregnancy by delaying ovulation, preventing fertilization, or altering the uterine lining. It is intended for occasional use and is not a replacement for regular contraceptive methods.

History and Development: Since its introduction, Postinor-2 has undergone significant development and gained approval in many countries worldwide. It has become a reliable option for emergency contraception due to its efficacy and safety profile.

Importance and Relevance: Postinor-2 plays a crucial role in preventing unintended pregnancies, especially in cases of contraceptive failure or unprotected sex. It offers women a second chance to avoid pregnancy and maintain control over their reproductive choices.

Mechanism of Action: Postinor-2 works primarily by delaying ovulation. If taken before ovulation, it can effectively prevent the release of an egg, thus preventing fertilization. It is less effective if ovulation has already occurred, highlighting the importance of timely administration.

Effectiveness: Postinor-2 is most effective when taken as soon as possible after unprotected sex. Its effectiveness diminishes with time, and it is not 100% foolproof. For women with higher body weight or BMI, its efficacy might be reduced.

Time Frame for Usage: Postinor-2 should be taken within 72 hours of unprotected intercourse for optimal effectiveness. The sooner it is taken, the better it works. Beyond 72 hours, other forms of emergency contraception, like the copper IUD, should be considered.

Usage Guidelines: Clear guidelines on indications, dosage, and administration of Postinor-2 ensure its proper use. It is crucial to follow these instructions and understand what to do in cases of vomiting or other complications.

Side Effects and Safety: Postinor-2 is generally safe, with most side effects being mild and temporary, such as nausea, fatigue, and menstrual changes. Rare but serious side effects should be monitored, and contraindications must be considered. Understanding interactions with other medications is also vital for safe use.

Frequently Asked Questions: Addressing common concerns about Postinor-2, such as its impact on future fertility, effectiveness during ovulation, and access, helps dispel myths and provide accurate information. Alternatives like the copper IUD and ulipristal acetate offer additional options for emergency contraception.

6.2 Final Recommendations

Based on the comprehensive understanding of Postinor-2 and its role in emergency contraception, several final recommendations can help individuals make informed choices and use this medication effectively and safely.

1. Timely Use: The effectiveness of Postinor-2 is highly dependent on the timing of administration. It should be taken as soon as possible after unprotected intercourse, ideally within 72 hours. Delays in taking the pill reduce its ability to prevent pregnancy.

2. Understanding Limitations: While Postinor-2 is a valuable option for emergency contraception, it is not 100% effective. Women should be aware of its limitations, particularly its reduced effectiveness during ovulation and for those with higher body weight or BMI. Alternative emergency contraceptives should be considered in such cases.

3. Awareness of Side Effects: Users should be informed about common side effects, such as nausea, headache, and menstrual changes. Knowing what to expect can help manage these side effects effectively. Any severe or unusual symptoms should prompt a visit to a healthcare provider.

4. Avoid Frequent Use: Postinor-2 is not intended for regular contraceptive use. Frequent reliance on emergency contraception can lead to more pronounced side effects and reduced effectiveness. Women who find themselves needing emergency contraception frequently should discuss long-term contraceptive options with a healthcare provider.

5. Seek Medical Advice: Consulting with a healthcare provider can provide personalized guidance on emergency contraception and help address any concerns or contraindications. Healthcare providers can also recommend alternative methods if Postinor-2 is not suitable.

6. Consider Long-Term Contraceptives: For more reliable and consistent contraception, long-term methods such as oral contraceptives, IUDs, implants, or injections are recommended. These methods provide ongoing protection and reduce the need for emergency contraception.

7. Educate and Inform: Increasing awareness and education about emergency contraception options, including Postinor-2, is crucial. Healthcare providers, educators, and community organizations play a vital role in disseminating accurate information and supporting informed decision-making.

8. Access and Availability: Ensuring easy access to Postinor-2 and other emergency contraceptives is essential. Pharmacies, healthcare clinics, and online platforms should make these medications readily available. Community programs and non-profits can help provide free or low-cost options for those in need.

9. Monitor Menstrual Cycle: After taking Postinor-2, women should monitor their menstrual cycle. While some irregularities are expected, a significantly delayed period warrants a pregnancy test. Any concerns about menstrual changes should be discussed with a healthcare provider.

10. Address Special Circumstances: Women in special circumstances, such as survivors of sexual assault or those with underlying health conditions, should receive tailored support and access to emergency contraception. Postinor-2 can be a crucial part of care in these situations.

FINALLY, Postinor-2 is a valuable emergency contraceptive that provides an essential option for preventing unintended pregnancies. Understanding its use, effectiveness, side effects, and safety considerations is crucial for informed decision-making. While Postinor-2 offers a reliable solution for emergency situations, it should not replace regular contraceptive methods. Educating women about their options and ensuring easy access to emergency contraception can empower them to maintain control over their reproductive health. Healthcare providers, educators, and community organizations play a vital role in supporting informed choices and promoting the safe and effective use of emergency contraception.

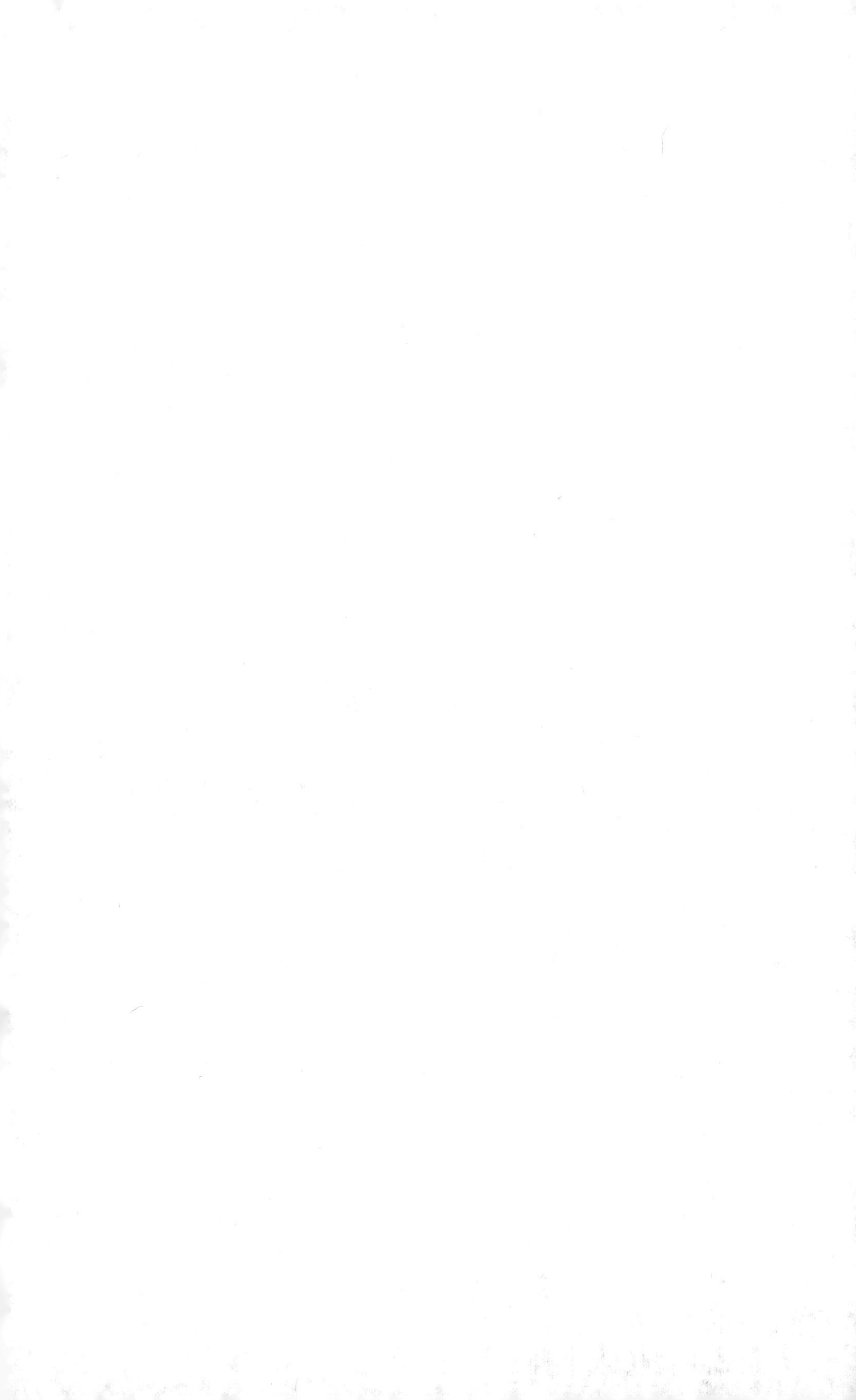

www.ingramcontent.com/pod-product-compliance
Lightning Source LLC
Chambersburg PA
CBHW051713250726

48653CB00007B/3014